The Spice of Life
Herbal Remedies From the Heart of Your Kitchen

By Mary Thibodeau

Copyright © 2016, by Mary Thibodeau. All rights reserved. No part of this publication may be reproduced, distributed, or transmitted in any form or by any means, including photocopying, recording, or other electronic or mechanical methods, without the prior written permission of the publisher, except in the case of brief quotations embodied in critical reviews and certain other noncommercial uses permitted by copyright law.

Disclaimer: This book is not intended as a substitute for the medical advice of your health care practitioner. The reader should regularly consult a physician in matters relating to his/her health and diet, and particularly with respect to any symptoms that may require diagnosis or medical attention.

Table of Contents by Herb

Introduction

Anise

Basil

Bay Leaf

Black Pepper

Cardamom

Cayenne

Celery Seed

Chile Powder

Chives

Cilantro

Cinnamon

Cloves

Coriander

Cumin

Dill

Fennel

Fenugreek

Ginger

Nutmeg

Oregano

Paprika

Parsley

Rosemary

Saffron

Sage

Tarragon

Thyme

Turmeric

Yellow Mustard Seed

Conclusion

Bonus eBook: *"12 Healing Herbal Recipes: Herbal Medicine the Delicious Way"*

INTRODUCTION

Most people have a cupboard or a rack filled with spices from all over the world. Herbs that originated in the far east or the middle east are now a mainstay in the kitchens of cooks across the globe. While sprinkling foods with these herbs has become commonplace, what has gotten lost is the knowledge of their medicinal powers.

The joining of herbalism and cooking is of great interest to me – as a practicing herbalist and holistic health maven, I am very fond of treating food as medicine, and vice versa.

To me it's a miracle to have the same foods that taste delicious also helping us with health conditions. Herbs and foods go hand in hand and this book was written with that in mind.

So get ready to see your spice rack in a whole new light. You'll soon be discovering the potent medicinal value that accompanies some of your best loved spices. You'll learn dozens of ways to use your culinary herbs for common first aid ailments. You won't need to go far to embark on your own journey with herbalism, it starts right in your kitchen.

How to Get the Best Spices

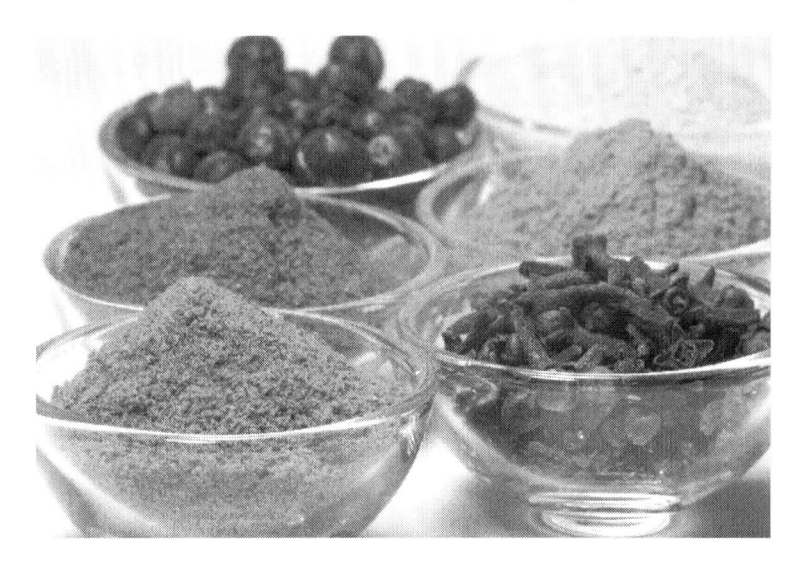

There are three main ways to obtain top quality herbs:

1-Natural Food Markets

This is my favorite choice because I can go into a locally owned store (in my case it's the Natural Living Center in Bangor, Maine; or John Edward's Market in Ellsworth) and buy organic spices at prices *far below* what you'd pay for commercial spices at, say Walmart. This I love. A way to save money and get better quality, it just doesn't get any better.

Each of these natural markets has a bulk herb area where you can bag up as much of any herb you desire, be it medicinal or culinary or both. The choices will astound you and the level of quality will probably surprise you. Organic herbs are fresher, their color and aroma is more vibrant, and they have not been sprayed or otherwise treated with preservatives or pesticides to lengthen their shelf life like most commercial herbs.

So in a nutshell, cheaper yet higher quality culinary herbs can be found in natural food markets. Bag up exactly how much you need, weigh it up, get your plu tag and add it to your grocery cart.

Most herbs (excepting maybe Saffron) are so cheap when bought this way you'll never go back to buying spices in your grocery store's baking aisle. It's like an herbalist's and cook's best kept secret.

2-Online

Of course you can find anything online. The benefits of buying your spices this way include convenience and a variety of choices so you can shop around. Still, it's important to try and purchase organic to ensure best quality. The downfall here is you must buy prepackaged amounts, but usually there are many options.

Also, it's good to know your source. A few reputable websites for culinary herbs online include Frontier Coop and Mountain Rose Herbs. I've used both companies over the years for both medicinal and culinary purchases.

3-Growing Your Own

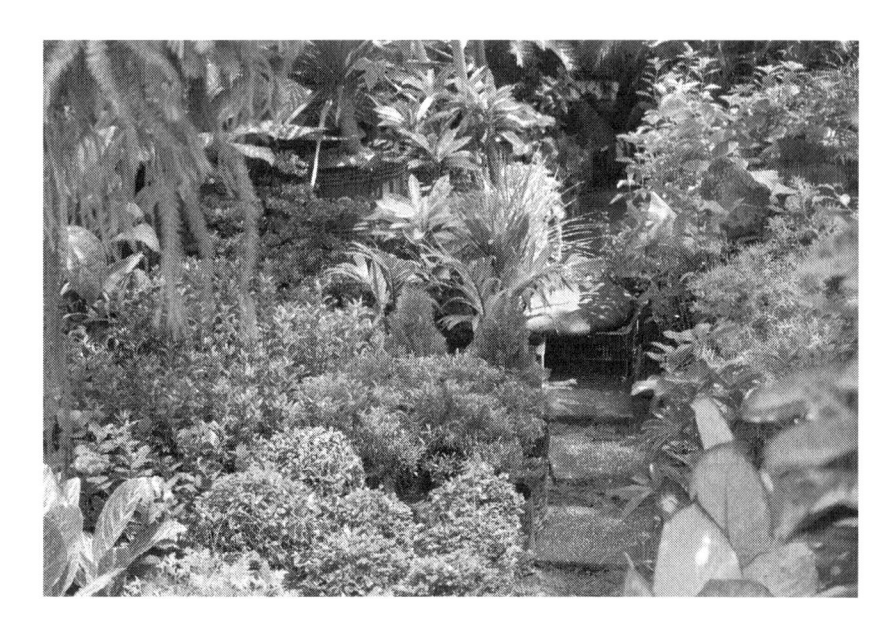

This is certainly a topic for a whole other book for sure, but I can tell you there is nothing better than taking a fresh cutting of herbs straight from your garden and putting them right into your recipes. The act of cutting enables you to do a little earthing (connecting with the earth's electromagnetic field), and you'll even experience a bit of aromatherapy in the process.

Some of the perennial herbs that I use regularly and that are easy to grow include Peppermint, Garden (or Rock) Thyme, Dill and Rosemary. There are about ten inches of fresh snow on the ground at this writing, but if I wanted to, I could dig down and get some fresh Thyme. It's been my experience that it simply cannot be killed!

Determining The Shelf Life of Spices

If you're like most people (myself included), there are herbs that are now in your cupboard that are quite possibly older than you are. Spices have a tendency to travel between generations and friends, apartments and cities.

You might inherit someone's spice collection, or you might move into a place and find some herbs left in the rack. Some you clearly remember buying, others you have no idea where the heck they came from.

If you're worried about the efficacy of a medicinal spice, or you're wanting to know if it still retains its flavor and medicinal value, there are two ways that I know of to determine their quality at any given time:

1-Color
Is it the same color as when you would buy a new supply of this herb? The color, when a spice is dried optimally, should be very close to the appearance of the fresh herb. If the herb's color is faded, so then are its medicinal and flavoring qualities.

2-Smell
This, I think, is the best way to determine whether an herb is still good or not. Does it smell as it should? If you're not sure, go to a natural food store and smell the herbs there! If the scent of a particular herb is very scant or negligible, it's probably time to toss it in the compost.

What to Expect

In this book, for each herb, I will outline the medicinal properties most appropriate for home use and offer at least one way in which that herb can be used for a first aid or general health ailment.

Special Note

Even though these herbs lay innocently in your kitchen ready for use in recipes and herbal remedies, they do represent powerful medicinal plants. Please consult with your healthcare practitioner before taking any herbal remedies. Many of the herbs can alter the potency and level of safety of over-the-counter and prescription medicines.

Anise

In the kitchen, Anise is mostly used for making sweets like Biscotti cookies and holiday candies, and in making specialty liqueurs. If you have some in your cupboard, just know that if someone has a gripping stomach ache, one of the quickest known ways to relieve it is to drink a cup of tea made with even just a few anise seeds.

Anise is a natural stomachic, a relaxant, a tonic and a carminative, working to quickly dispel gas and even treat colic.

One of the oldest herbs in recorded history, Anise has also been used traditionally to treat upper respiratory diseases. In addition to its gastrointestinal benefits, this herb also has antiseptic, diaphoretic (sweat inducing) and expectorant qualities. Chewing on one little seed can also instantly freshen your breath.

Basil

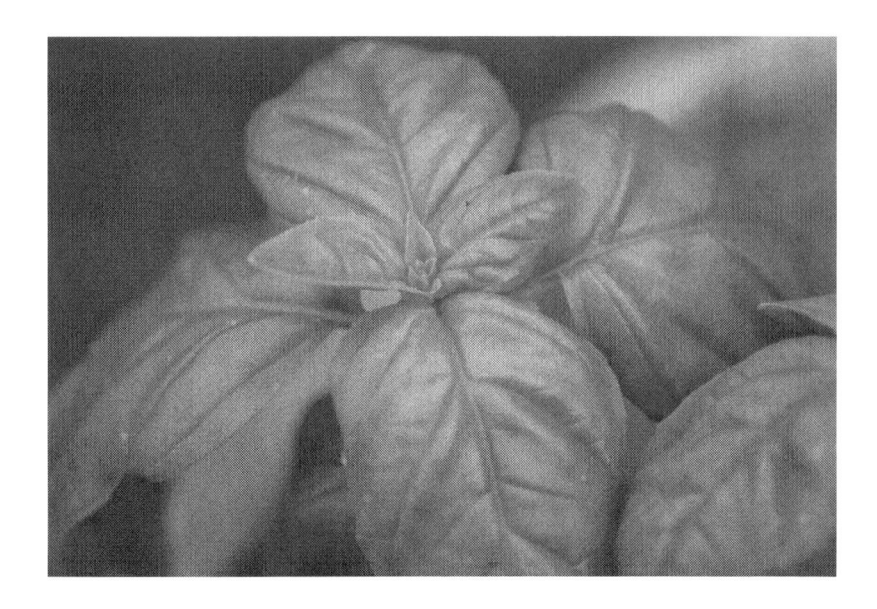

Quite possibly one of the most loved herbs, a bottle of dried basil probably now graces the spice rack in most kitchens worldwide. Its uses are almost infinite, availability is a given, and its healing actions are many.

Basil has numerous medicinal properties including anti-inflammatory, antioxidant and antibacterial while also packing a nutritional punch with minerals iron, calcium and manganese, and vitamins A, K and C as well as folate.

Used for thousands of years, Basil nowadays can almost always be found in any Italian recipe and in many soups. I love to add the dried herb by the tablespoonful to my homemade marinara sauce and vegetable soup.

Since most of us have some dried Basil in the kitchen, we can easily use it to help in normalizing blood sugar levels simply by having a cup of Basil tea every day. Another useful way to take Basil as medicine is to do a steam inhalation of the tea, which can reduce headache pain and anxiety. This tea can even be added to a bath for an exotic stress reduction treatment.

I know a lot of us enjoy using fresh basil as well, and since it is so easily grown or bought locally, I'd like to include a recipe here - a way to make your medicine taste really good!

RECIPE: Quick & Easy Basil Pesto

Ingredients:
2 cups fresh basil leaves (found in most U.S. produce departments)
½ cup walnuts
3 garlic cloves
½ cup olive oil
1 T lemon juice
3 T nutritional yeast (found in natural food markets and/or online)

Directions:

In a food processor or high speed blender, grind up the basil, walnuts and garlic. Drizzle the oil over this mixture slowly as you blend it more. Then add lemon juice and nutritional yeast and blend again.

While many folks like to mix pesto in with pasta, there are many other ways to use this delicious, nutrition-packed herbal treat. Try using it as a pizza topping instead of marinara sauce. It also makes a great dip for veggies and rice crackers, can be baked into a bread recipe and is often used as salad dressing.

Bay Leaves

Historically, Bay Leaves are known throughout Greece and Rome as a symbol of honor, as seen in the crowns of laurels worn by VIP's in ancient civilizations (it's scientific name is Laurus Nobilis).

Nowadays, you will find this culinary herb mostly used in soups and stews. By looking a little more closely at this famous herb you can find a few surprising details about its effectiveness in treating a variety of ailments.

Just a simple cup of Bay Leaf Tea acts as a mild diuretic. Its astringent qualities are beneficial in assisting in the drying up of secretions and reducing excess sweating in cases of fever.

Externally, Bay Leaf has traditionally been used by herbalists because of its antimicrobial properties and its ability to accelerate wound healing. In this case a tea can be cooled and directly applied, or a clean cloth may be soaked in tea and place on the wound.

Bay Leaf has been found to positively affect blood sugar levels in those with Type 2 Diabetes - only 1 gram of the herb taken per day over time showed significant improvement in levels of blood sugar, cholesterol and overall insulin function.

Black Pepper

We use black pepper so much in the West that it's uncommon to even think of it as an herb - but in reality it's quite useful medicinally. The great thing is that there probably isn't a household without it!

Long used in Ayurveda, Black Pepper is considered a digestive herb, in that it stimulates digestive enzymes helping to metabolize food. When you taste even just a tiny amount of Black Pepper, a release of hydrochloric acid, needed for protein digestion, is automatically released.

Pepper is also a heating herb, as you probably well know, and this fact along with its antioxidant content makes this herb great at drying up mucous in cases of upper respiratory congestion. A simple yet soothing cold medicine can be made with honey and Black Pepper.

Caution: Large amounts or doses of Black Pepper are not recommended. This may inhibit the metabolism of other prescription or over-the-counter medicines.

Cardamom

I've been a big fan of Cardamom ever since my sister made me my first ever cup of Yogi Tea. The aroma and flavor of this exotic herb is uplifting in itself, not to mention all of its healing potential.

I could probably write an eBook just about this versatile little seed pod, but will try to sum things up here. Cardamom is known for its mood enhancing abilities and in some cultures is considered an aphrodisiac. It's also widely known as a cancer preventative with its volatile oils and high level of antioxidants and minerals.

For the cardiovascular system, Cardamom can normalize blood pressure and inhibit excessive clotting. Recently studies on Cardamom's effects in urinary tract infections have shown positive results.

As with many of these kitchen herbs, Cardamom is also a digestive tonic, helping to increase the movement of food through the intestines.

To enjoy the flavor and feel the power of Cardamom, try a cup of Yogi Tea. The herbs in the recipe below are quite strong, if you feel you have a tender stomach, add more milk to cut the mixture and even make it a little creamier:

Yogi Tea Recipe

Ingredients:
1 Quart Water
8 Cloves
8 Cardamom Pods
8 Black Peppercorns
1 Teaspoon Fresh Grated Ginger (or powdered)
1 Cinnamon Stick (or a teaspoon of powder)
1 Tea Bag, Black or Green Tea
Optional Ingredients: Milk of your choice & Honey to taste

Directions:
Simmer the herbs in water for 30 minutes
Add tea bag and optional ingredients
Let steep for 10 minutes and enjoy!

Cayenne

Cayenne is one of my favorite herbs to have around to add to soups, curries, hummus and guacamole. In fact, it has so many medicinal uses in addition to adding a hot flavor to anything, that if you could have just one spice in the kitchen, this would be a perfect candidate.

Not only is Cayenne a digestive, heart and kidney tonic when taken internally, but its very nature is warming and stimulating, making it a great winter herb to add into soups and stews. Any recipe calling for black pepper will taste better with cayenne, in my opinion.

Externally, as in an infused oil or made into a salve, Cayenne gives relief to those suffering joint or muscle pain.

Tradition tells us the same as current medical studies - Cayenne acts as a circulatory stimulant, a cardiovascular tonic if you will, a restorative for the digestive system, even positively affecting ulcers, and as an anti-cancer herb.

Celery Seed

Unlike many spices, where the seeds that are used for culinary purposes taste far different, and often better or more exotically flavored than the original plant, celery seeds are pretty cut and dry - they make whatever you are flavoring them with taste like celery, only the flavor is a bit longer lasting. So they often work best where you want a celery flavor - pickles, salads, chutneys, sauces, stir fries and pasta dishes.

Used as an Indian Ayurvedic herb for thousands of years, celery seed was traditionally prescribed for colds, flus, joint pain, liver issues, water retention and digestive complaints. In current times, drawing on that knowledge in addition to recent studies, Celery Seed is used extensively as a reliever of menstrual cramps.

By reducing inflammation and muscle spasms while calming nerves and regulating blood pressure, Celery Seed eases the cramping during menstruation. It's also used medicinally as a natural diuretic.

Caution: Because of its effects on cramps, blood pressure and inflammation, it should not be used during pregnancy.

Chile Powder

The reputation of Chile's uses in a pain relieving capacity has been growing over the past few decades. When used in external applications (always in an oil or ointment of some kind, never applied directly!), Chile powder can be very helpful in relieving nerve pain, muscle pain and arthritis.

A simple oil can be made by steeping 2 teaspoons of dried chile in the oil of your choice for 30 minutes, warming but never boiling. Cool and use as a massage oil.

Hint: Using almond or grapeseed oil makes a less oily oil, if that makes any sense! Basically these oils are more effective at being absorbed into the skin. Olive oil can certainly be used as it is less expensive and has its own nutritive properties, and that is what I usually use.

Internally, Chiles represents one of the major circulatory stimulants available. Its warming, sweat inducing and circulatory improving properties contribute to its positive effects on the heart. Chiles also are high in Vitamin C and are anti-bacterial, making them yet another immunity supporting herb. Use them in your favorite spicy dish.

Caution: Do not use internally in excessive amounts, or it can be damaging to your organs.

Chives

Not surprisingly, since they are in the same family as onions and garlic, Chives can be used in numerous medicinal ways, just like their cousins.

In Medieval times this plant was hung in homes to ward off evil. Or maybe, because of its antibacterial properties and Vitamin C content, Chives were helping to stay deadly viruses or the plague. Either way, it was commonly seen in homes and had a reputation for lifting melancholy.

As an appetite stimulant and digestive tonic, Chives can be readily added in fresh or dried form to soups, salads or main dishes. They also have been shown to help promote low blood pressure and are high in folic acid.

In the garden, if you like growing herbs, Chives make a great border plant and are effective in repelling pests like aphids. They also grow like a typical garden weed and require minimal care.

Cilantro

Traditionally used for culinary purposes in flavoring soups, pesto, salsa and many main dish recipes, Cilantro is now gaining popularity for both its nutritional and medicinal value. The more I write and study herbs, the more I understand this connection between good food and health. To me, herbs represent powerhouses of nutrition that our bodies want and need.

While many cultures consider the term Cilantro to mean the same as Coriander, in the U.S. (erroneously or not), when we say Cilantro we're talking about the leaves of the plant, and when saying Coriander, we're talking about the seeds.

So back to Cilantro (the greens), this little herb has actually been used in chelation therapy, or in the removal of heavy metals in humans. Its natural cleansing abilities, potent antioxidant constituents and blood purifying properties make it one of earth's best natural detoxifiers.

Nutritionally, Cilantro is one of the highest herb forms of Vitamin K, which is now being studied for its role in inhibiting the neuronal damage in the brains of Alzheimer's patients. It also is packed with minerals including iron and manganese and antioxidant Vitamins A and C.

Adding a handful of fresh or a tablespoon of dried Cilantro to your salsa, hummus, black bean recipe or soup will add delicious flavor and a high level of phytonutrients.

Cinnamon

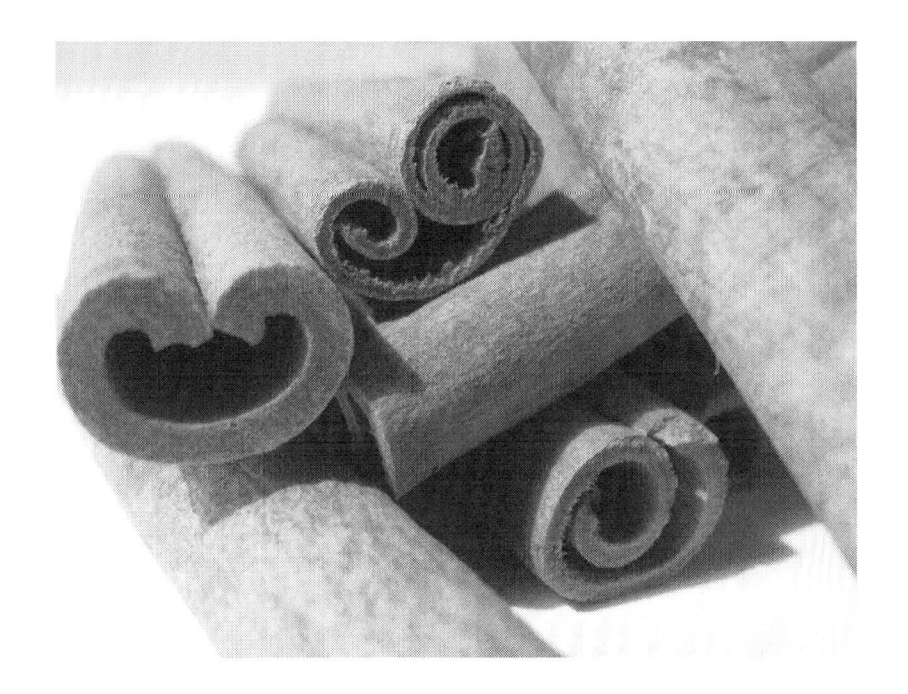

Westerners are accustomed to having cinnamon in some form almost daily, from breakfast cereals, oatmeal and muffins, to delicious desserts and specialty beverages. Most kitchens are going to have a steady supply of cinnamon flowing.

While ground cinnamon bark has numerous medicinal uses (like most herbs), the one I'll focus on here is its power in relieving menstrual cramps. I've written pretty extensively about cinnamon in my other books (i.e. Immune System Boosters) and I try to always offer added value and not repeat myself for my readers.

Cinnamon has been helping women with menstrual cramping for centuries and has recently been studied for not only its effects on relieving cramps, but also how it contributes to decreasing the amount of cramps and pain over time. With its abilities to reduce clotting, its anti-inflammatory actions, while toning the uterus and urinary system, Cinnamon has been shown to be effective in treating not just menstrual cramping, but other associated PMS symptoms, such as back pain and nausea.

It's as easy as making yourself a cup of cinnamon tea for the 5-6 days preceding your period. Simmer one teaspoon of ground cinnamon in water, and add milk and sweetener of your choice.

Cloves

This is one kitchen spice you may have heard of in the context of its healing powers. Its use as a pain reliever especially for toothaches has been documented since before 200 B.C.

A small clean cloth soaked in a strong cloves decoction (1 teaspoon per cup of water, simmered for 30 minutes and cooled to room temperature) can be directly applied to the affected area of distress. This dental herbal remedy preceded by far modern dentistry and has been used extensively by traditional herbalists worldwide.

It also makes a quick and easy remedy to prepare and use at home. Quick and easy is important when someone is suffering from tooth pain.

An oil can also be made and applied repeatedly. Use 2 teaspoons of crushed cloves in 1 cup of olive oil (or other oil of your choice) and heat, never boil, for 20 minutes. The oil will stay on the affected area for longer and may offer a more lasting relief than an infusion.

The plant itself possesses analgesic (pain relieving) and mood enhancing properties and is, in general, a warming carminative herb, meaning it is a soothing tonic. So while the toothache is being treated, the rest of the body is also enjoying a gentle digestive enhancer and an energizing boost.

Coriander

Coriander, the dried seed of the plant most Americans refer to as Cilantro, was recommended by Hippocrates in Ancient Greece as a tonic herb. High in Vitamins A, Folate, B6, C and K, and minerals iron, calcium and manganese, Coriander has long been used in Indian, Chinese, Italian, Greek and Egyptian cuisine.

With a warm, nutty, orangey flavor easily brought out by grinding and adding to your cooking oil (most Americans buy this herb already ground), Coriander doesn't just make a nice, spicy addition, but also packs in powerful anti-inflammatory, antiseptic and antifungal properties making it perfect for any fungal or inflamed skin issue (i.e. eczema, athlete's foot, etc.) and internal parasites. It's also been used as a preventative for food poisoning.

To make an easy, flavorful oil for marinating, or as a salad dressing, simply combine 1 teaspoon of coriander seeds (ground) with 1 clove of minced garlic, juice of ½ lemon and oil of your choice, I recommend olive. Let sit for a few hours or warm for 10 minutes before cooking with, or cooling and adding to your salad.

Cumin

As with many culinary herbs, as I'm sure you will realize after reading this book, Cumin not only adds a spicy, delicious flavor to rice dishes, curries, chilies and soups, but it also packs in super phytonutrients. Cumin is high in minerals iron, copper, selenium and zinc, and Vitamins E, A, C and B-Complex.

Traditionally it's had many uses as a natural medicine including as an arthritis remedy, a protector from memory loss, an immune response enhancer, a digestive tonic and a blood sugar regulator. This latter use has continued into modern times as lab tests have confirmed this effect.

You may already be using Cumin on a regular basis without knowing it - most Chile spice mixes, taco mixes and curry spices have lots of Cumin in them. If you're not already cooking with it, you can begin now to add it to any recipes you like to have spicy, or you can simply make a tea with 1 teaspoon per cup of water and enjoy Cumin's ability to improve digestion by enhancing the production of enzymatic secretions.

Dill

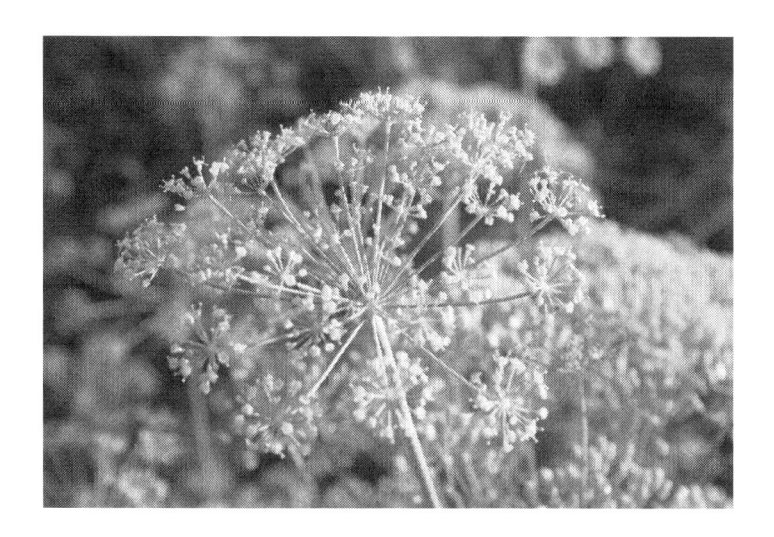

Even as an herbalist, I often think first of pickles when hearing the word 'dill'. But this herb, which I just started growing last year in my own herb garden, way outshines its reputation in flavoring preserved veggies. In fact, not only does this herb pack a high vitamin content, but it also is one of the premier herbs in reducing flatulence and colic.

Coming from the Norse word, dilla, meaning "lull to sleep", Dill is such a powerful digestive stimulant and tonic, that it can quickly ease stomach cramps while quieting nerves and promoting sleep! Who knew?

Dill has also been used by herbalists in relieving headaches brought on by overeating and food allergies (think migraines) as its cooling carminative and indigestion relieving properties help that messed up meal you just ate exit the arena while you feel calmed and restored.

If you have a baby with colic in the house, try soaking a washcloth in a strong dill tea and letting the babe suck on the cloth. Not only can it help with the painful cramping, but may also act as a sleep aid: win, win.

Fennel

This herb, with its unusually sweet flavor, is a safe and gentle remedy to use for infants, elderly persons and those with compromised immune systems.

A tea with Fennel can be used as an eyewash for pinkeye and sties, as its antiseptic and anti-inflammatory powers work effectively here. The ancient Greeks and Romans knick-named it the "Herb of Sight" and it was used regularly for clearing up vision problems, cataracts and milky eyes.

As a carminative (gas relieving), a digestive tonic, and a nervous system stimulant, Fennel treats the weak and the strong by easing stomach cramping while also promoting mental alertness.

While the seeds are what's usually used in herbal preparations, the bulbs may also be used medicinally.

This is one herb that can be used freely with children and the sick. Lastly, it is also a galactogogue, promoting mother's milk when the tea is drunk by a lactating woman.

Fenugreek

There are numerous accounts of Fenugreek Seeds having positive effects on blood sugar levels for diabetics, and it is said to slow the absorption of sugar in the intestinal tract and stimulate the production of insulin. This herbal remedy is commonly used in the West as a diabetes supporting supplement.

Personally I like to consider this a Goddess Herb. It tastes syrupy sweet, is an aphrodisiac, calms PMS symptoms and promotes milk flow in lactating moms. It's also chock full of minerals, vitamins, fiber and, unusually for an herb, calories.

Caution: Not to be used during pregnancy, since it may cause uterine contractions.

Ginger

I could write a whole book about the benefits of Ginger and if you've read my other books, I'm sure you seen mention of this awesome king of herbs.

For this book I will focus on its abilities in relieving nausea - be it from morning sickness, motion sickness, sea sickness, migraines, surgery recovery or chemotherapy, Ginger is nausea's butt kicker.

It accomplishes this with its anti-inflammatory actions coupled with it promotion of gas elimination and soothing action in the intestinal tract. Countless of studies have been done to prove this ability and many have been focused specifically on finding a remedy for motion sickness and morning sickness, two very common ailments in today's world.

This is my all-time favorite herb to make tea with. Usually I use the fresh herb chopped and decocted, but if I don't have any on hand, powdered works, too.

Anti-Nausea Tea Recipe
Using 1 teaspoon Powdered Ginger (or 1 tablespoon fresh grated) per cup of water, boil the herb for 10 minutes, strain, and add a bit of maple syrup and lemon to taste, pure deliciousness and comfort on a cold dark winter morning.

Nutmeg

If you're stressed out while cooking supper for the family, open your cupboard and take out the nutmeg. This amazing herb, the seed of a beautiful, tropical evergreen tree, lurks in your spice rack, probably only making an appearance for the apple pie you make for Thanksgiving.

Historically used in Roman emperor coronations as a fumigant to clean the streets before the royal procession, this highly aromatic herb targets nervous disorders and digestive problems simultaneously. A digestive tonic especially effective in gastritis or just plain old gas pain, Nutmeg also relieves nausea and is a potent antidepressant.

As a bonus, Nutmeg is also high in minerals (among them copper and iron) and antioxidant Vitamins A and C.

Caution: Only a small amount should be used as large doses can be toxic.

Put a pinch in your rice dish, oatmeal, soup or stir fry. You can also make a tea, but with Nutmeg alone the flavor may be a bit strong for some. Adding some cloves, cinnamon and ginger will make for a delicious hot drink to nurse while you're cooking that dinner under undue stress.

Oregano

From the mint family, Oregano was documented as being used in Ancient Greece for everything from convulsions to heart failure. Its high concentrations of antioxidants and phytonutrients have been studied extensively in recent years and the essential oil of Oregano is often touted as one of the most powerful antimicrobial and antibacterial substances available.

The information about Oregano Oil is usually pertaining to ingesting the diluted essential oil. While I'm fully aware that many herbalists have centered their businesses around this type of practice, I am not convinced of the safety. I've had a two experiences with ingesting essential oils - one was when my 3-year-old put his mouth on the top of an opened bottle of cinnamon essential oil. His mouth only touched it before I snatched it away, but he was in such distress I had to call Poison Control (coating the inside of the child's mouth with olive oil was what they recommended and what worked immediately). The other time, I had a persistent, long term lung ailment and as a last ditch effort, I drank water with 2 drops of Oregano Oil. My natural reaction told me all I needed to know about ingesting essential oils - my body hated it and wanted to repel it instantly! It was the foulest taste I have ever experienced. And I eat a lot of wild things!

Essential Oils, while powerful healers when inhaled, are essentially vapors, not meant to be digested, and most wise women herbalists will agree with me on this point.

So back to Oregano, you don't have to suck down a watered down, potentially hazardous essential oil to reap the benefits this little herb has to offer.

By making a tea or an infused oil with Oregano, you are preserving an herbal medicine that can be used on any fungal problems, athlete's foot, dandruff, and intestinal parasites. The tea can be added to your bath or even your shampoo bottle. You may already be using this herb when making Italian dishes, so feel free to add more to your recipes, preferably toward the end of cooking time so the medicinal qualities don't get cooked out.

Paprika

A lot of Americans are familiar with using Paprika as a festive splash of color on deviled eggs and potato salads. Made from select varieties of peppers, and revered in Hungary for adding smoky, spicy or savory flavors to just about anything, this vibrant herb can easily be included in your diet by adding it to your cooking oil, salsa, soup, hummus, chili, potato dishes, curry, etc.

What I never knew until delving into the research available on this herb, is that it's an excellent remedy for skin problems. With its high concentration of Beta Carotene and B6, along with potent antibacterial actions, adding Paprika into your diet or applying it directly to your skin as in a mask, can help improve your complexion.

It may even restrict the amount of melanin produced in your skin thus limiting age spots and it can help prevent wrinkles. The recipe below will leave your skin with a super soft glow.

FACIAL MASK RECIPE

Ingredients:
1 Avocado
1 Tablespoon Honey (Agave Syrup is a vegan alternative)
1 teaspoon ground Paprika

Directions:
Mash together, apply to face and leave on for 15-20 minutes (don't worry if some gets in your mouth - it's delicious!)

Parsley

The next time you see a sprig of fresh parsley on your plate as a garnish, feel free to eat it then and there - it's probably by far the healthiest food available on your plate!

Now while most of the kitchen herbs I'm writing about in this book are in their dried, spice-rack-ready form, I will include information here about fresh parsley because it is both easy to grow and sold in most every Western produce department.

One of my favorite nutritional herbs, just a half cup of fresh Parsley will provide a solid level of every known Vitamin excluding B12 and Vitamin D. It's especially high in Vitamins K, A, C and Folate and also contains good amounts of minerals iron, copper and calcium.

By adding Parsley daily or even weekly into your meal plans, you are providing a chemoprotective food that may neutralize carcinogens. It's been shown in lab studies to inhibit the growth of tumors, especially in the lungs.

Parsley tastes great in pesto, soups, marinara, salads and just about any cooked or raw dish. It's best to use as fresh as possible, so if adding to cooked recipes, put it in at the end. I've found that a bunch of fresh Parsley bought at the grocery store will last a couple weeks in my crisper drawer in the fridge.

Rosemary

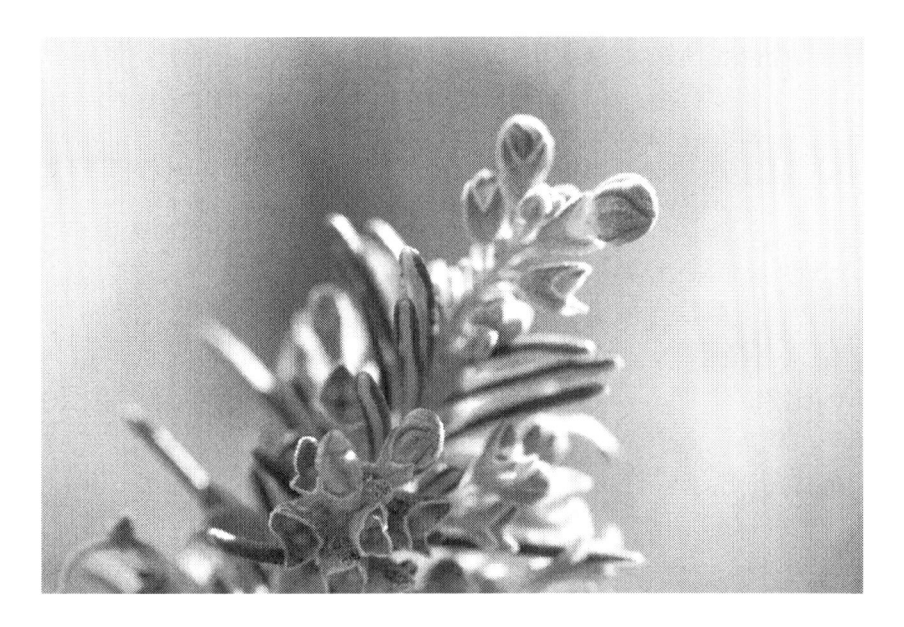

I am not much of an indoor plant person - I'd rather be out in the garden or foraging - but one herb I do keep inside is Rosemary. I keep it in my kitchen mainly for two reasons. First of all, here in Maine it won't survive outside, so I bring it in during the cold months.

Secondly, while in the house, it makes the perfect reminder for me to keep hydrated in wintertime because of the dryness of heating systems. Rosemary, which loves hot and dry air, will wilt quickly without careful and copious watering whenever it's cold enough for the heat to be on. I think the same goes for humans and I find the more I pay attention to proper hydration (really getting those 8 cups per day), the healthier I am overall.

The third reason why Rosemary makes such a good houseplant, is that it's easy and super delicious to cut a few leaves, chop them up and put them on a baked potato or in rice. A quick, easy to way to feel invigorated by Rosemary's effects.

Taken over time, Rosemary has been shown in studies to improve memory and fight cancer.

Saffron

Everything about Saffron seems exotic to me. In America, you usually only find it the most expensive restaurants, where it adds taste, aroma and a gorgeous yellow tint to rice dishes and other entrees.

At $20 per gram, I won't spend too much time here, who can afford that? But its medicinal properties have long been recognized and used in folk medicine for relieving asthma, as an expectorant, analgesic and sedative. In fact, these last two pain relieving qualities are probably why even today in Morocco, some mothers traditionally rub the gums of their teething babes with a gold ring coated in honey and Saffron.

Caution: Lethal in large doses!!!

Sage

In Medieval folklore, Sage was used by midwives in stopping premature labor, but during this time it was also considered a "cure all," especially for curbing excess passions. Nowadays we might just call this female feistiness and I know of no herbalists who are recommending the cutting out of passions!

In modern times, Sage's reputation as a hair growth stimulant is just now starting to gain momentum. But this herb's main use is in drying up excess secretions. It would be helpful in treating night sweats, hot flashes, bleeding sores, and congestion.

One way to clear up stuffed up sinuses is to soak a cloth in a strong dose of Sage tea and lay down with it on your forehead. It also makes a great gargle when you feel a tickle in your throat and a cold coming on. But this gargle you can drink and as an added bonus, you can even enjoy some inner calmness and clarity as it also acts as a muscle relaxant and a nervine.

This might be an herb that men would be interested in using, and not just because of the hair growth stimulation actions, but because Sage has a definite masculine scent.

Caution: If lactating, regular dosing with Sage can dry of the flow of breastmilk.

Tarragon

This aromatic herb, while highly prized in France and used as a gourmet herb around the world (and much less expensive than Saffron!), represents another perfect herb for toothaches. Like Cloves, mentioned above, Tarragon contains eugenol, a substance that has a numbing effect on the mouth.

But instead of making an oil or a compress, like you do with Cloves when treating dental pain, you can simply chew on a few of the Tarragon seeds and enjoy the analgesic effects. It's also a mild sedative and antidepressant.

Caution: Do not use when pregnant.

Thyme

There are a lot of reasons why I love thyme; one is that I have it growing in my yard and no matter if it's the darkest, coldest month of winter, I can still dig through the snow and find some fresh thyme leaves - even here in Maine!

This herb is so versatile and can be used for numerous ailments from external treatments like easing rashes, to internal applications as in calming the nervous system, and on and on.

For first aid purposes, I think its strength lies in its antimicrobial, antifungal and antibiotic properties.

When you feel a sore throat starting and you know a cold or something worse is coming, make a strong cup of Thyme Tea, using a half cup or so of the herb to 2-3 cups of water. Gargle with it, only don't spit out the tea! Swallow some of nature's antibiotic and continue on doing this right through any sickness.

For colds, flus and other respiratory ailments, Thyme acts as an expectorant, has a calming effect on respiratory spasms and fights germs. Just what you need when a cold or sickness is coming on.

Turmeric

If you follow natural health news, you've probably already heard about this kitchen herb and its amazing capabilities. One of its constituents, curcumin, is the real showstopper packing in one of mother nature's top anti-inflammatories.

While its powers have long been known by herbalists, recently many studies have been done comparing Turmeric to pharmaceutical anti-inflammatories and the results showed that the Turmeric effects were similar - only no adverse side effects were found.

A chronic low level of Inflammation has now been identified as a major player in most chronic Western diseases, including cancer, heart disease and Alzheimer's. This is where Turmeric comes in and provides us with a super powerful anti-inflammatory and antioxidant right out of the kitchen cupboard.

While this spice is normally used in curries, mustards and cheeses, it also can favorably affect the circulatory system, improve brain function, protect against free radicals and help relieve the pain of arthritis. You can enjoy a daily cup of Turmeric tea by adding 1 teaspoon of the herb to a cup of water, simmer for ten minutes and drink. It also tastes good with ginger and cinnamon.

Yellow Mustard Seed

You may be surprised to see this herb here. In fact, you may never have even considered it an herb at all! It's not just for hot dogs and pickles; mustard seed has stimulating and warming qualities and is chock full of phytonutrients, minerals and vitamins.

As a circulatory stimulator, mustard seed can be used to allay neck and shoulder pain by using a mustard pack. The heat created and the stimulating effects can slow down throbbing pain and grant genuine relief.

A mustard pack may be used by grinding 2 tablespoons of the seed, adding a bit of warm water and flour to make a paste. Then wrap the poultice in a clean cotton cloth (that you don't mind getting stained) and apply directly to the source of discomfort.

Conclusion

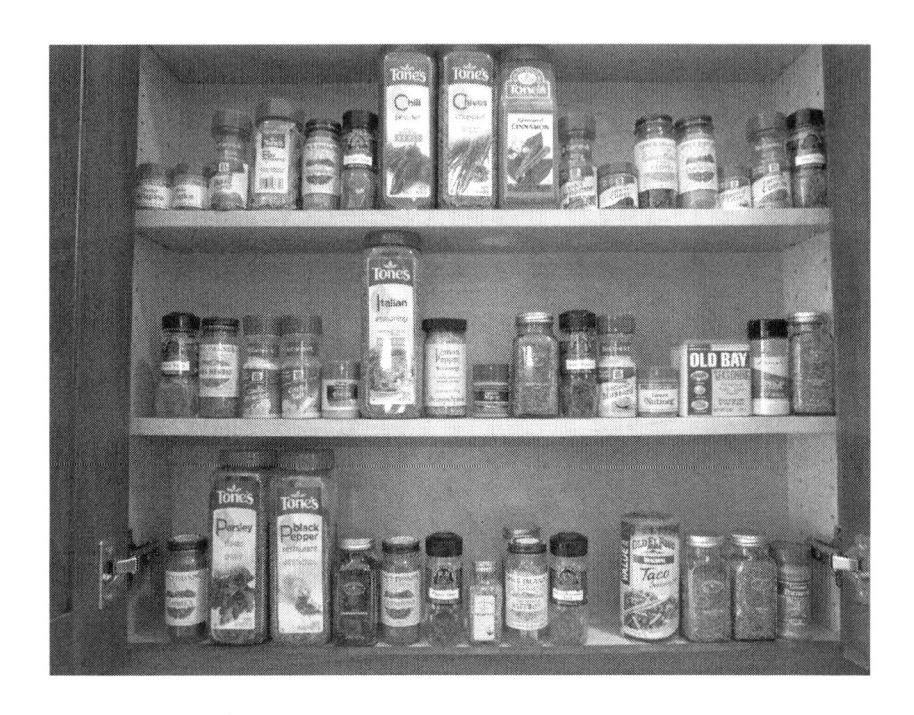

Many times when we're throwing together a new recipe for dinner or a special occasion, we're focused on getting the correct ingredients and amounts. We're worrying about missing something or overcooking or not having it rise properly.

How often do we stop and take in the aroma of an herb like Anise or Cilantro? How wonderful it is to have these amazing spices within our reach in the hearts of our home.

After cooking three meals a day for three children for over a decade, I sometimes just want to avoid the kitchen altogether. But having a cupboard full of potent medicinal herbs can sometimes help to spark the culinary artist in even the most kitchen-adverse people.

When we are cooking with herbs and spices, whether it be something as simple as black pepper, or an exotic herb like Saffron, not only are we creating a delicious dish for ourselves or for friends or family, we are also enabling ourselves to give medicine in the most beautiful of ways - through food. We can make a delicious soup or a spicy salsa or an aromatic cup of tea and soothe not just our hungries, but our bodies as well.

I hope that the next time you walk into your kitchen and open your cupboard or look at your spice rack, you'll see not only a means to cooking appealing foods, but also a way to heal our bodies.

Culinary spices have more than one purpose - it's time to embrace the medicinal qualities of these herbs and know that they are there for us and our families in times of need.

Thank you for reading and please be sure to leave your honest feedback in a review under Mary Thibodeau at Amazon.com

12 Healing Herbal Recipes
Herbal Medicine
The Delicious Way

By Mary Thibodeau

Copyright © 2015, by Mary Thibodeau. All rights reserved. No part of this publication may be reproduced, distributed, or transmitted in any form or by any means, including photocopying, recording, or other electronic or mechanical methods, without the prior written permission of the publisher, except in the case of brief quotations embodied in critical reviews and certain other noncommercial uses permitted by copyright law.

Disclaimer: This book is not intended as a substitute for the medical advice of your health care practitioner. The reader should regularly consult a physician in matters relating to his/her health and diet, and particularly with respect to any symptoms that may require diagnosis or medical attention.

Table of Contents

Introduction

Mango Cilantro Salad

Passionflower Tea

Carob Flax Fudge

Super Hummus

Creamy Mushroom Tomato Soup

Pickled Garlic

Cold Curried Rice Salad

Dandy Green Smoothie

Spicy Guacamole

Chaga Coffee

Herbal Marinara

Basil Pesto

Conclusion

Free Gift

More Books by Mary Thibodeau

Introduction

I hope that you've been wanting to learn about cooking meals and snacks for yourself and your family while enjoying the many medicinal properties that herbs have to offer. Because that's what this book is about. I started studying herbalism right around the same time I became interested in herbal nutrition, about sixteen years ago as of this writing.

I have come to understand that food and medicine are intricately related and that the line between health and diet is really not a line at all. What you eat, what you put into your body three to five times a day, actually represents your best chance at positively affecting your health. By bringing a focus to the medicinal and nutritive herbs in our diets we are maximizing our chances of long term wellness.

Mango Cilantro Salad

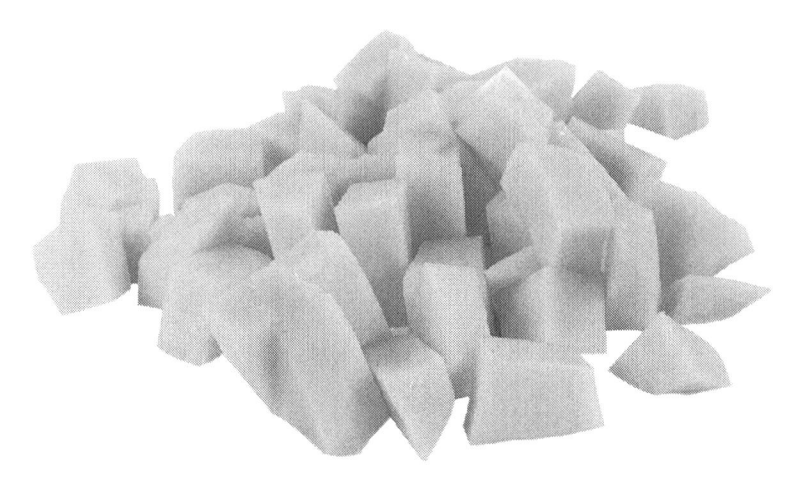

Salads should not be something you HAVE to eat; they should be a work of art and sumptuous. How the heck else are we going to want to eat one every day, which everybody knows we should be doing? This recipe will help ease salads into your daily routine, because it makes for a spectacular visual (beautiful food = good), is super yummy and has a high level of nutrition with medicinal actions helping you on the side.

Ingredients:

2 teaspoons balsamic vinegar

2 teaspoons fresh lime juice

1 teaspoon maple syrup

3 Tablespoons olive oil

1 large Mango, peeled and chopped

1 medium cucumber, peeled and chopped

½ red onion, chopped finely

1/3 cup fresh cilantro chopped

Dash of salt

Directions:

Whisk together first 4 ingredients (the dressing) until emulsified, then add all other ingredients, coating well. Serve immediately or chill for later use.

Featured Herb: Cilantro

Traditionally used for culinary purposes in flavoring soups, pesto, salsa and many main dish recipes, Cilantro is now gaining popularity for both its nutritional and medicinal value.

This powerful herb has actually been used in chelation therapy, meaning in the removal of heavy metals in humans. Its natural cleansing abilities, potent antioxidant constituents, and blood purifying properties make it one of earth's best natural detoxifiers.

Nutritional Summary for Mango Cilantro Salad:

Nutritionally, Cilantro is one of the highest herb forms of Vitamin K, which is now being studied for its role in inhibiting neuronal damage in the brains of

Alzheimer's patients. It also is packed with minerals including iron and manganese, and antioxidant Vitamins A and C. To give you an idea of just how amazing Cilantro is, check out the additional nutritional information below:

(Based on daily recommended values for the salad as a whole)

242% Vitamin A

222% Vitamin C

82% Vitamin K

67% Vitamin E

73% Copper

55% Vitamin B6

53% Folate

35% Manganese

29% Potassium

10% Iron

10% Calcium

Passionflower Tea Blend

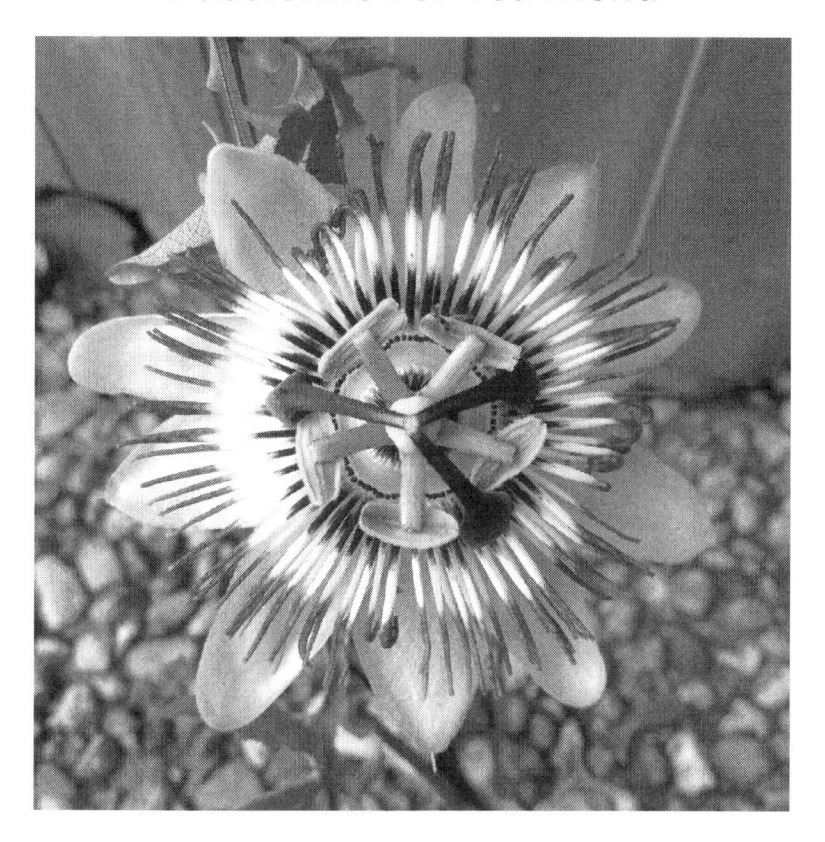

This, to me, is luxury defined. A gorgeous plant, translated into a warming, soothing and tasty drink to sip alone or share with a friend. The art of making an herbal tea alone is relaxing, and in this recipe you will feel the calming benefits almost immediately upon your first sip.

Ingredients:

1 tsp of Dried Passionflower herb

1 tsp of Dried Chamomile herb

1 tsp of Dried Peppermint herb

(*if using fresh herbs, use 1 Tablespoon)

Directions:

Boil 8oz water

Place herbs in a tea infuser or tea ball (alternatively if you don't have an infuser, you can strain the herbs before drinking)

Pour boiling water into the cup with the herbs and infuser inside. Cover if possible and let steep for at least 15 minutes.

Featured Herbs: Passionflower, Chamomile & Peppermint

I used this recipe here because these herbs together are so potent and effective at reducing stress and anxiety. Together they also work to ease upset stomachs, and soothe irritation in the throat and lungs during colds and the flu.

It's the perfect blend to keep around the house in times of upheaval or excitement. This passionflower tea also makes the perfect sleepy time tea and has been used traditionally to cure insomnia.

Nutritional Summary: Passionflower Tea

Together, these three herbs will support your body with minerals including copper and manganese. It also contains trace B Vitamins. Their main importance here is not in the nutritional arena, though the tea acts as a digestive aid helping to better digest other foods.

Carob Flax Fudge

This is a fabulous dessert; easy, quick and super nutritious. There's no baking involved; it's basically melting a few things together, adding dry ingredients and packing it down into a cake pan, then throwing in the fridge to set up. Chocolate and processed sugar are both Migraine triggers for me, so this is the one of the few desserts that I get to enjoy, and I always bring it to family and holiday get-togethers so there is an option that not only is spectacularly yummy, but that also contributes to my vegan dietary needs.

There are many ways to change up the recipe and I've listed some alternative ingredients to give you an idea of that. Keep in mind this is a high protein/high (good) fat dessert with a lot of calories, so it doesn't make a good everyday food – but it's perfect for special occasions. It works especially well with people who have gluten, dairy or egg allergies.

Ingredients

1 cup peanut butter (or any nut butter)

1 cup maple syrup (or honey)

1 cup carob powder (cocoa powder could be substituted here)

1 cup coconut (the more the better!!!)

½ cup ground nuts (pistachio are my favorite, but peanuts are great, too)

1 Tbls ground flax seed (ground sunflower seeds also work well)

1 tsp ground cinnamon

Directions

In a medium to large sized pot, heat and stir the maple syrup and peanut butter together until smooth. It just takes a couple minutes. Add all the other ingredients and stir in well, a big spoon works well for this. Then, scoop out and flatten down into a baking pan or cake pan, until the brownies are about ½ inch or a little less. Flatten and even it down with a spatula and then chill. If you need the fudge ready quickly, freeze for 30 minutes, otherwise, let it chill in the fridge for a couple of hours. Enjoy!!

Featured Herbs

Who would have thought that you could eat a dessert that had so much medicinal content! The cinnamon in my fudge recipe adds antibacterial and anti-inflammatory properties, while the flax seeds provide protection again breast and ovarian cancer.[i]

Nutritional Summary

You would not even believe the nutrition that is packed into this recipe. With one or two servings, you'll receive the full range of healthy proteins and amino acids, differing amounts of all major vitamins and minerals (with the exception of Vitamins D and B12) and quite possibly, the best known sources of essential fatty acids.

Super Hummus

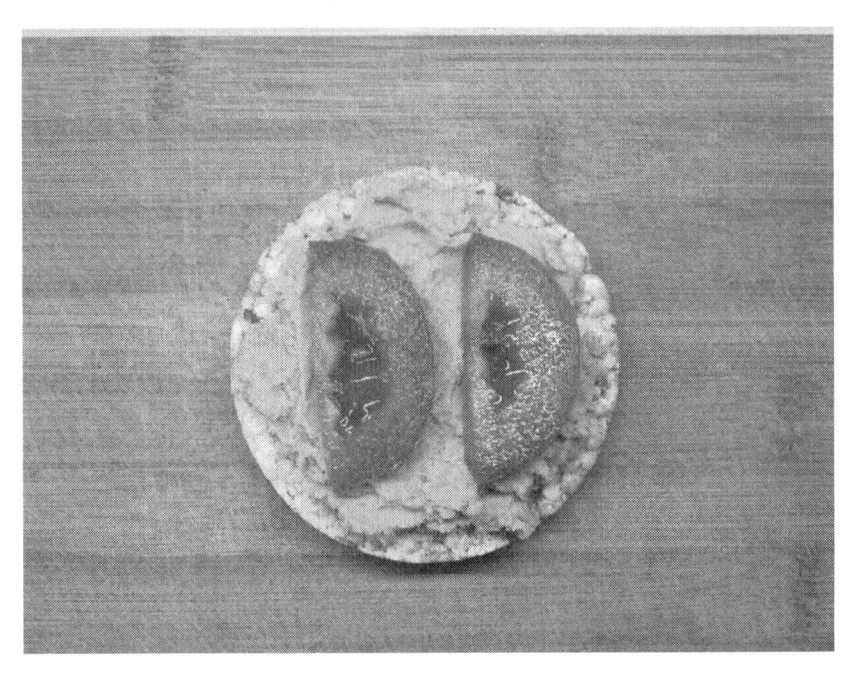

Hummus is a satisfyingly filling and delicious snack or meal accompaniment that is also highly nutritious. Add in some extra garlic and cayenne, you have a healthy heart and immunity boosting side dish. This hummus is so good I could eat it alone without a problem!

Ingredients

2 T Olive Oil

¼ chopped red pepper, sautéed in scarce amount of oil

2-3 cloves of roasted garlic (see directions; raw garlic is good, too, but overpowering for some people)

2 cans of chickpeas (garbanzo beans)

¼ cup of Tahini

Pinch of cayenne

1 T lime juice

Desired amount of salt – depending on your tastes. I like minimal salt in this recipe because the roasted garlic gives so much flavor. I feel salt is barely even needed at all.

Directions

To begin, roast an entire bulb of garlic by this method: take one bulb and slice the very bottom off, so the cloves are exposed. Place them in a baking pan exposed-side up and drizzle the open end with olive oil. Cover loosely with foil and bake at 400F for 30 minutes. When done, the garlic will be soft, squishy and awesomely scrumptious.

While the garlic is roasting, sauté the red pepper in a bit of oil until soft. When pepper and garlic are done, combine them with all other ingredients in a high speed mixer (I use a Nutri-bullet) adding a bit of water for consistency.

Featured Herbs

Garlic again! The immunity powerhouse, only this time excruciatingly tasty. Roasting the garlic brings out the sweetness and preserves much, but not all, of garlic's immunity boosting actions.

Nutritional Summary

This is a great source of protein and healthy fats, as the ingredients offer ample amino acids and EFA's. It's also abundant in antioxidant Vitamins A, C and E, and is heavy on the minerals, most notably Copper, Manganese, Phosphorus, Selenium, Zinc and Iron.

Creamy Mushroom Tomato Soup

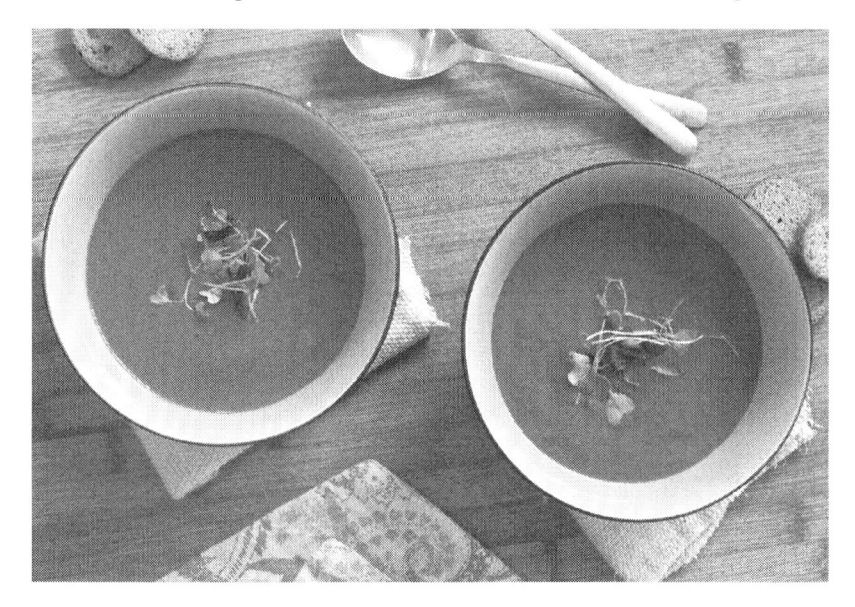

If you have kids, or feed multiple people with varying tastes or dietary needs, then this may be the recipe for you. I have been making this same soup for years and years and not one of my kids has ever complained. And with three, all with unique ideas of their own, this is a feat if there ever was one for me in the kitchen. The only complaints that ever came was when I made the soup without a certain ingredient, or tried something different. So I try to keep it the same and we eat this soup about once per week, year-round. I think it pleases everyone because it's a creamy tomato soup and those are hard to pass up. What I love is that it's loaded with healthful herbs and fresh veggies. The way I make it, it's dairy free and gluten free.

Ingredients

2-3 medium sized tomatoes, sliced

1 can tomato sauce

1 Portobello mushroom, chopped

1 medium sized potato, chopped with peel on

1 onion, diced

¼ red pepper, diced

Optional: chopped zucchini (my kids like both with and without, for us it depends on the season)

Fresh herbs if available: 1 Tbs each of Thyme, Oregano & Basil

Dried herbs are also fine: 1tsp Thyme, 1Tbs oregano & Basil

½ cup frozen non-gmo Corn

½ can Garbanzo beans (or black beans or other bean)

Directions

Start this out by sautéing in a soup pot the onion, mushroom and pepper until the onion is translucent (at this point the sweetness comes out). Then add the chopped potato and tomato slices (and optional zucchini) and enough water just to cover everything.

Simmer this mixture for 15 minutes, making sure the potatoes are soft. Then puree the mixture before putting back into the soup pot. It will be super thick and creamy from the mushroom and the potato starch. Add the can of tomato sauce and enough water for your desired amount of soup, the less you add the thicker it will be. Add all of the herbs and heat to boil.

Add rice pasta (for gluten free, or whatever pasta strikes your fancy) and simmer, stirring frequently for 15 minutes (or however long your pasta takes to cook). Before serving, add frozen corn and/or garbanzo beans and heat just a bit. I add the corn and beans at the end because only one kid likes beans in his soup, and I do aim to please!

Featured Herbs

I've found that in my travels as a holistic food freak and herbalist, that there are quite a few items that are on the threshold – are they food or are they herbal medicine. In this soup there are several crossover ingredients: Portobello mushrooms, onions and red peppers. Portobello mushrooms are nutrient dense and also viewed as powerful anti-inflammatory agents. Onions are super high in flavonoids and in the herbal world are considered one of nature's best "drawing" medicines. And red peppers, the number one food source of Vitamin C, are actually well known for their anti-inflammatory and anti-oxidant effects.

Nutritional Summary

In addition to the herbal wonders this recipe offers, with the mushrooms, tahini and garbanzo beans you also reap many nutritive benefits, including a wide array of B-Complex and anti-oxidant vitamins, and a high content of minerals including copper, potassium, iron and calcium.

Pickled Garlic

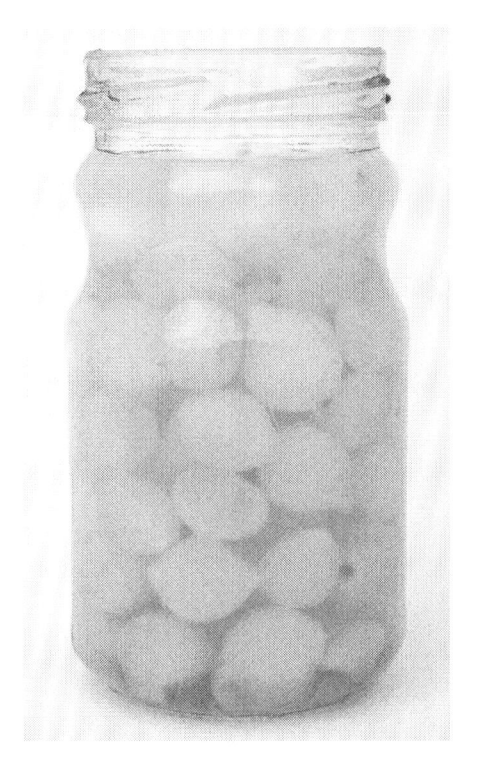

I probably can't even explain how much I love this recipe. The biggest reason is that you can get all the super antibacterial actions of raw garlic, but it doesn't taste like raw garlic! Instead it gets sweeter and sweeter in time, and makes having a daily or even weekly dose of 'nature's penicillin' easy and great tasting.

Before I knew about pickled garlic, I would occasionally eat raw garlic. Either just by popping a raw clove or by chopping and mixing with orange or grapefruit juice. Neither way an attractive snack! I love roasted garlic, but once you cook it down this way, you lose a lot of this herb's goodness.

Pickling the garlic allows you to eat practically raw garlic and actually enjoy it instead of being horrified. That's why I love it.

Ingredients

Raw, peeled, whole garlic cloves. Try not to nick them as you peel them. Any nicked cloves will still be fine to eat, but they will brown a bit at the nick's site. Doesn't make a difference taste-wise or medicinally, only aesthetically. Use as many as you want, if it's a small, 4oz ball jar, you can fit around 10 whole cloves, depending on the size.

Apple Cider Vinegar

Honey or Maple Syrup to taste

Directions

If you get this going on July 1st you'll have your pickled garlic ready for the cold weather and change of seasons. It takes about twelve total weeks. Simply fill your jar with the whole, raw cloves, fill to the top with apple cider vinegar, and try to cover all the cloves with the liquid. Cap tightly and let sit in dark warmth for about six weeks. After this time period, strain and keep half the liquid. Take this liquid and add an equal amount of sweetener, warming the mixture gently on the stove. Pour over garlic in the jar, cap tightly again and let sit another six weeks, or even longer. It will get softer and sweeter as time goes. After this, it's ready to eat as is, or spread over some nice bread or even added to a soup directly before serving. It's yummy sweet garlic, with the raw benefits!

Featured Herbs

Garlic goes solo in this recipe. Historically, garlic has been used for thousands of years that we know of. Early Egyptian records found garlic in the pyramids. In 18th century France, grave diggers were using it in hopes of warding off the plague. And in both World Wars, garlic was given to soldiers to prevent gangrene.

In today's world, garlic supplements are often taken by those with cardiovascular disease and to boost immunity. Some studies even suggest taking garlic acts as a cancer preventative.

Scientists have found that by taking garlic over a 12-week period during the cold and flu season, that the likelihood of coming down with a cold significantly decreases, and the symptoms that do occur are less severe and last a shorter duration.[ii]

Eating a clove pickled in this way may give even more benefits, since the product is preserved well and more fresh than what you might get in buying the dried supplement.

Nutritional Summary

Eating two pickled cloves will give your body not only immune supporting medicine, but will also add manganese and other trace minerals, and Vitamin C. This recipe is more medicine than food, but still tastes great.

Cold Curried Rice Salad

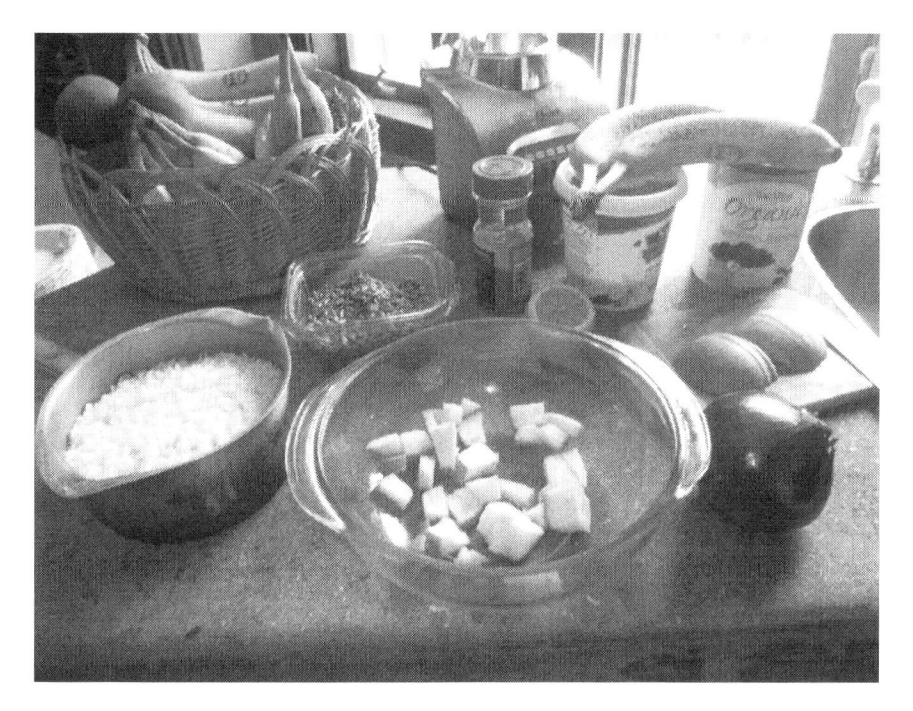

This my favorite potluck dish to bring. I'll be honest; this recipe was never a favorite with my kids, but it was always loved by other moms. It's festive, unique and is not only tasty, but filling and nutritious, too.

<u>Ingredients</u>

2 cups cooked brown or white rice

¼ red onion

½ cup coconut (or other) yogurt (or mayo)

2 Tbls curry powder (or less or more, this would make it rather spicy.)

2 bananas chopped

1 green apple diced, with peels

¼ cup sunflower seeds

½ - 1 cup of raisins (depending on how sweet you want it)

Salt to taste

Bit of lemon juice

Optional: Coconut shreds for garnish

Directions

While your rice is cooking, get a mixing bowl and squeeze some fresh lemon juice into it. Then chop the apple, onion and bananas and add them to the bowl, mixing with the lemon. Add all other ingredients except the coconut garnish and mix well, adding more yogurt if needed, or salt or raisins for taste. Let this mixture cool in the refrigerator until the rice is cooled down, then mix all together. Chill well and sprinkle on coconut before serving.

Featured Herbs

A good curry blend will include a mixture of many, top herbal medicinals, including coriander, turmeric, cumin, fenugreek, and chili peppers. Let's take a look quickly at each herb:

Coriander: High in Vitamins A, Folate, B6, C and K, and minerals iron, calcium and manganese, Coriander has long been used in Indian, Chinese, Italian, Greek and Egyptian cuisine.

Turmeric: While its powers have long been known by herbalists, recently many studies have been done comparing Turmeric to pharmaceutical anti-inflammatories and the results showed that the Turmeric effects were similar - only no adverse side effects were found.

Cumin: Cumin Seriously packs in some super phytonutrients. This traditional herb that has been used for millennia, is high in minerals iron, copper, selenium and zinc, and Vitamins E, A, C and B-Complex.

Fenugreek: There are numerous studies showing the positive effects Fenugreek has on blood sugar levels for diabetics. It is said to slow the absorption of sugar in the intestinal tract and stimulate the production of insulin. Fenugreek is also, in my opinion, a Goddess Herb. It tastes syrupy sweet, is an aphrodisiac, calms PMS symptoms and promotes milk flow in lactating moms. It's also chock full of minerals, vitamins, fiber and, unusually for an herb, calories.

Chile Peppers: This herb represents one of the major circulatory stimulants available. Its warming, sweat inducing and circulatory improving properties contribute to its positive effects on the heart. Chiles also are high in Vitamin C and are anti-bacterial.

Nutritional Summary for 1 serving (8 total in recipe)

This salad, let me tell you, just about has it all. All Vitamins except D and especially high in B5, B6 and E. It also contains healthy amounts of all the major amino acids and minerals along with your omega fatty acids.

Dandy Green Smoothie (With a Zing!)

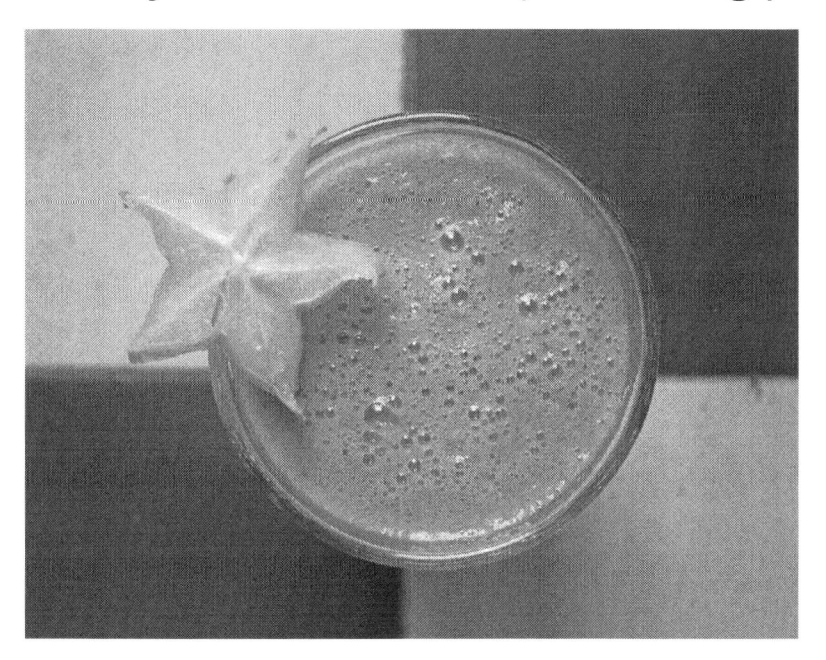

This is what I consider the perfect way to start your day; sort of a pre-breakfast. While some green smoothies are protein based, filled with ground seeds and nut milks (and those are great, too!), my concoction is in it for the greens - and making them tasty! Forgive me if I assume, but I do think we could all use some more fresh greens in our diets, I know I do!

Ingredients

1 cup fresh dandelion greens (believe it or not, most U.S. grocery stores stock this in the produce department.)

1 cup fresh spinach

1 cup fresh or frozen mango

1 cup fresh or frozen banana (fresh or frozen depends on whether or not you like your smoothies cold or room temp – your choice!)

Juice of 1 lemon

1 T freshly grated ginger (the "Zing")

Splash of maple syrup to taste

½ to 1 cup of water (depending on your type of mixer, food processors may need more water, while high powered 'ninja-like' devices will blend well without much liquid.)

Directions

Mix it up and enjoy!

Featured Herbs

Ginger. What herbalist or foodie doesn't love ginger?! A crossover food that enjoys high popularity as both food and medicine, ginger provides numerous medicinal properties including (but not limited to), analgesic (pain relieving), anti-inflammatory, antifungal, antibacterial, immune system boosting, anti-clotting, anti-nausea and digestive tonic.

Nutritional Summary

Well, in this smoothie you have your fruits, banana and mango, filled with potassium, antioxidant Vitamins and all around deliciousness. Then you've got your greens. With Dandelion Greens you get off the charts Vitamins K and A, half of your daily Vitamin C and ALL KNOWN MINERALS. Add in some spinach and you again get rich with Vitamins A and K, while also getting about 30% of your daily Folate along with a nice spread of healthy proteins.

Spicy Guacamole

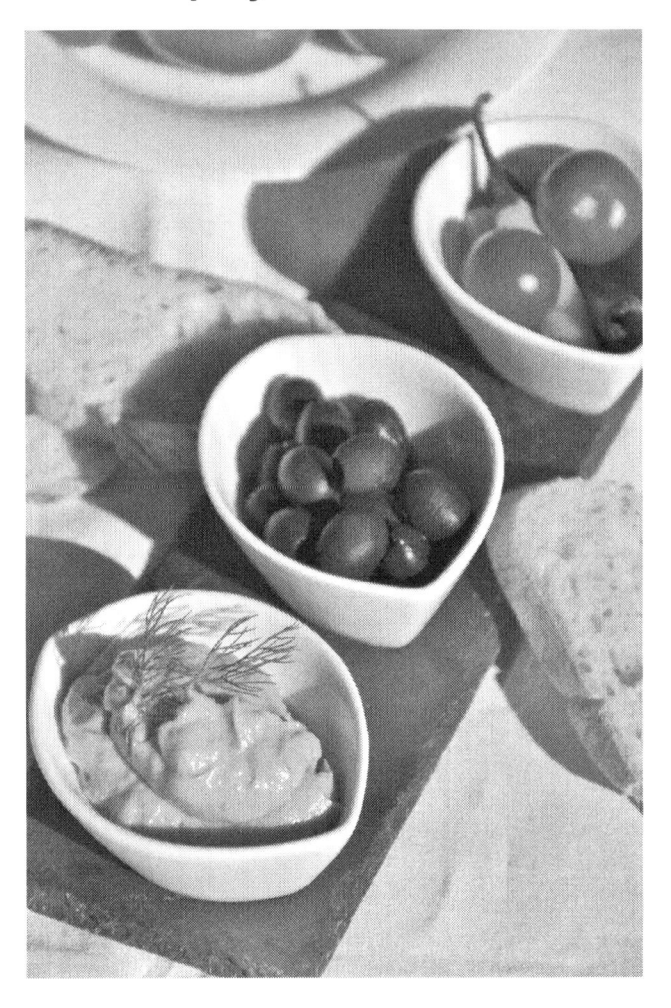

This is going to be by far the simplest recipe in this book, but sometimes the simple foods are the most luscious. And this one has been one of my favorites for a long time.

The first time I ever ate an avocado was in my early twenties when I lived out in the Phoenix area. I was instructed to simply sprinkle the cut avocado pieces with a little lime juice and eat it just like that. I loved it that way and still enjoy eating it like that sometimes. But my fav is to add a little pizazz and a little creaminess, as you'll see below. It's super quick to make and best when eaten fresh. Dip your corn chips, veggies or bread in your spicy guac, or add it to your sandwiches, salads or even use it as a pizza topping.

Ingredients

1 Avocado scooped, seeded and mashed
1 pinch of Cayenne (or 2 or 3 if you like it hot)
1 teaspoon of fresh lime juice
2 teaspoons of coconut (or other) yogurt

Directions

Puree or otherwise process all ingredients until smooth and creamy. For a party or family gathering simply double or triple the recipe, just adding ½ extra pinch of Cayenne per extra avocado.

Featured Herbs

Cayenne has numerous medicinal uses, including as a GI tract, heart and kidney tonic. It's very nature is warming and stimulating, aiding the circulatory, cardiovascular and digestive systems. Some studies have even suggested that Cayenne positively affects ulcers and helps prevent cancer.

Nutritional Summary

While Cayenne, Lime and Avocado all have Vitamin C, it's the Avocados that are packing in the most nutrients in this recipe. With over 25% of your daily C, they are also high in Vitamins B5, B6 and K and contain solid amounts of all nutritive minerals plus healthy fats and protein.

Chaga "Coffee"

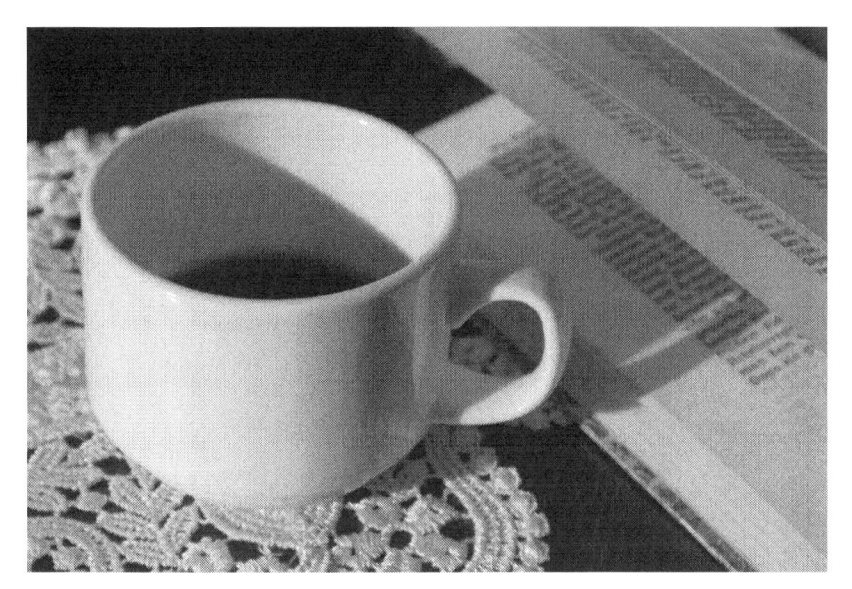

I first heard about Chaga about 4 years ago from another Mom at my kids' school. We were all standing in the hall, waiting for the bell to ring and our kids to be dismissed for pick up. Many of the other people waiting had bad colds and that week lots of kids had been out sick.

So this is what we were gabbing about when she happened mentioned that she doesn't get colds as long as she drinks her Chaga in the winter time. I was like, what? She even promised to bring some in so I could check it out and she offered to show it to me where she finds it along the Maine coast. I still haven't gotten out there yet with her, but plan to, and I've certainly been on the look-out in my area (with no luck yet!). She did bring in a big bag for me and I took to it right away.

Chaga does not taste like coffee, nor does it give you the caffeine burst, let me first make this disclosure. But it tastes smooth and earthy plus it gives you a multitude of medicinal benefits.

Ingredients

Grated, dried Chaga, the same amount as you would put in to brew coffee

Directions

Brew it like you would your normal pot of coffee. You can also decoct it to get even more medicine out of this wonder shroom. Decocting is simply simmering for 20 to 30 minutes, straining and drinking. Either way, you get to drink a rich, dark brew that treats you better than coffee.

Featured Herbs

Chaga has been shown in studies over and again to stimulate the body's ability to heal itself. This mushroom contains betulin, which controls metabolic disorders, and betulinic acid acts as anti-tumor agent. Chaga also directly aids the immune system by adding a multitude of antioxidants and acts as a potent anti-inflammatory. Inflammation is often the source of chronic disease, so supplementing with Chaga helps you to shore up your system so chronic disease doesn't take over your life.

Nutritional Summary

Touted as nature's most nutritionally dense tree growth, Chaga rises above all other fungi! Containing most B Vitamins and one of the highest sources of Pantothenic Acid in nature, Chaga is also significantly high in riboflavin, niacin and minerals copper, calcium, zinc and iron.

Herbal Marinara

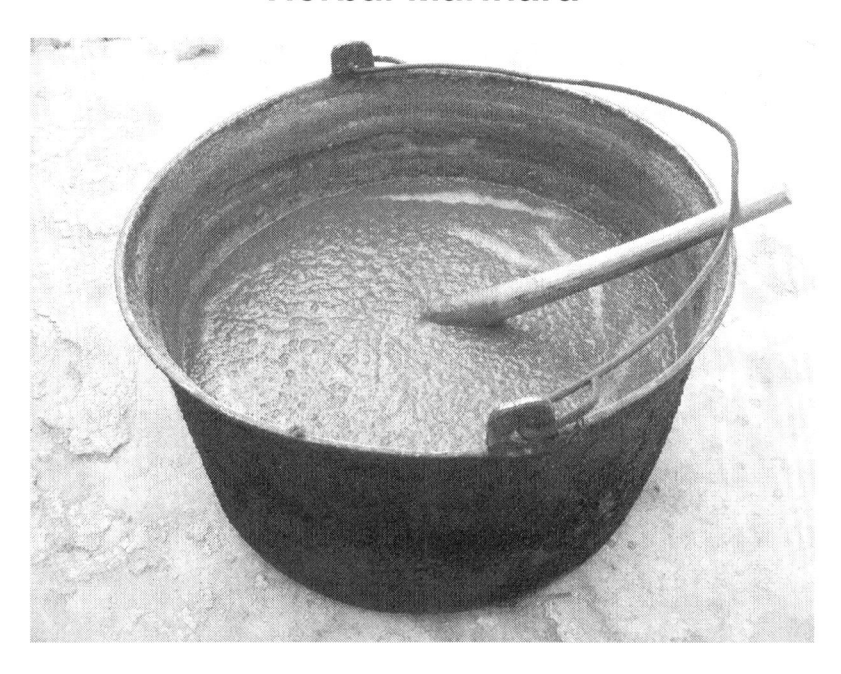

I don't like to brag, by my marinara recipe is so good, sometimes my kids ask for some in a bowl to eat plain with a spoon after it's been simmering for a while and is nice and hot. We even have a name for this, the kids call it, "Soo."

Not only do we used it for pasta (always better the 2nd day) but we've also been known to use it for dipping homemade bread sticks and corn chips.

What they don't know, and probably don't want to know (YOU try living with a health nut Mom for years on end!), is that this sauce is filled with super healing herbs and spices, along with ample nutritional benefits.

Ingredients

1 large onion

1 tablespoon of olive oil

1 red or green pepper

1-2 cups mushrooms (I like to buy the prepacked mix of oyster, shitake and mini bellas that they have in my grocery store)

1-2 cloves of garlic

2-3 medium sized tomatoes

3 cans of tomato sauce (or 2 large cans)

1 can tomato paste

Teaspoon of maple syrup

Sprinkle of cinnamon

2-3 tablespoons dried oregano

1 tablespoon dried basil

1 teaspoon dried thyme

Pinch of cayenne

Bit of salt to taste

Directions

Saute the onion, pepper and mushrooms until nice and tender. Add the garlic and saute a few moments longer. Put this mixture into a food processor with the chopped tomatoes (**note, my kids do not like a lot of chunks, if you like the chunky marinara style, forgo the food processing step, and just add in the chopped tomatoes and continue with the next steps).

Add mixture back to the pot and put in the remaining ingredients. Simmer for at least a few hours. The longer, the better. It's even yummier if you wait until the next day to eat it.

Use it to top your favorite pasta, and it also makes the perfect pizza sauce.

Featured Herbs

This recipe is chock full of herbs, the Italian seasoning group of herbs basil, oregano & thyme, along with a little cayenne, cinnamon and even a good amount of red pepper and mushrooms. If I gave you a complete rundown of all the ingredients in my Herbal Marinara, it could be a book all on its own. I'll try to summarize:

Basil, Oregano and Thyme all have antibacterial, antifungal and antiviral properties. Basil also is considered a nervine and carminative (gas relieving), while Oregano adds anti-oxidant support, anti-inflammatory properties, cancer fighting abilities and is great in treating upper respiratory diseases. Thyme chimes in with its antiseptic and anti-parasitic actions along with being anti-rheumatic.

Then you've got the mushrooms weighing in with their antiviral, antibacterial and antifungal support. And this really is the short version, since this is a recipe book!

Nutritional Summary

I tried to screen shot the nutritional breakdown of this recipe but it was too huge to fit in an eBook. Now I'm sounding like Donald Trump! I plugged in all the ingredients into Cronometer.com and this recipe hit every vitamin, EFA, mineral, amino acid and macro nutrient with the exception of Vitamin B12. Highlights include vast amounts of Vitamins A and C, B5 & B6, as well as high amounts of Copper, Iron, Manganes and Potassium. This is good food, period.

Basil Pesto

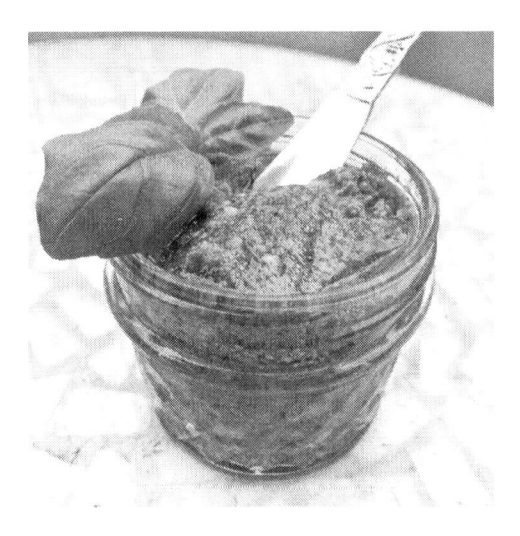

Pesto does not just have to be eaten with pasta; it can be baked into bread, added to soup, used as a dip for crackers or bread, as a pizza topping, salad dressing or even as a spicy addition to your omelet. What's extremely important is that pesto can disguise the taste of raw garlic very nicely and even sumptuously. So not only are you getting all that fabulous basil herb, but you're getting your shot of natural antibiotics as well.

What I love most about this recipe is that is the ultimate FAST FOOD. It literally takes 5 minutes to make and you're ready to enjoy a fantastic herbal delight.

Ingredients

1 bunch of fresh basil pesto, or two cups chopped

½ cups pine nuts (cashews or walnuts also work well)

½ cup oil (or cut the fat in half by using 1 avocado instead)

4 large cloves of garlic, chopped

Teaspoon of lemon juice

Pinch of cayenne

Salt and pepper to taste

A bit of almond milk (or other milk) if needed in blending

Directions

This is the best part: Just throw it all in to a food processor. I have a Nutri-bullet that works well. You may have to stop a few times to add a little liquid and scrape the sides to make sure everything is blended smoothly. And that's it - keep refrigerated and use prolifically!

Featured Herbs

Basil is the superpower house herb as far as I'm concerned. We've already mentioned in the previous recipes how this herb fights bacteria, provides anti-oxidant support and relieves gas. But did you know that Basil also represents one of nature's finest nerve tonics, as well as having fever reducing, cough expectorant, kidney and heart tonifying and insect repelling abilities?

Nutritional Summary

While the nuts and olive oil (or avocado) give you some nice healthy fats, garlic packs in the immunity boosting punch while Basil offers a high content of Vitamins K and C plus calcium, iron and EFA's.

I have only really touched on the surface on the powers of Basil, believe it or not. It's also very easy to grow in the garden and I can tell you, there is nothing better than pesto made with your own, fresh garden Basil!

Conclusion

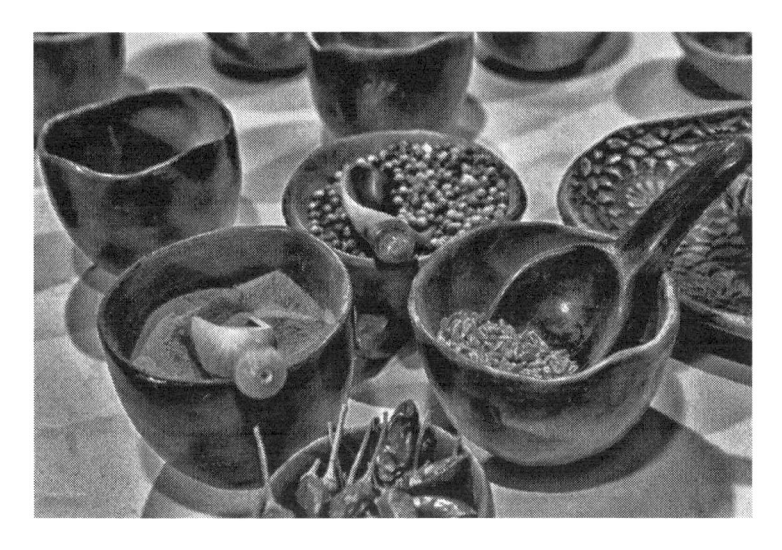

When you look at the culinary herbs in the picture above, most people associate those images with spices. By now you are aware that the spices that grace our kitchens are also potent medicinals. Welcome to my world!! This books represents many of the staple foods that I prepare for my family in keeping healthy – the delicious way!

I hope you've enjoyed this recipe book and that you're looking forward to trying some tasty yet healthy treats! This book was inspired by one of my subscribers who made the suggestion after reading "The Spice of Life: Herbal Remedies from the Heart of Your Kitchen," and soon this book and that one will be available together in a paperback version for everyone's kitchen.

Please feel free to leave an honest review under Mary Thibodeau at www.Amazon.com.

Also, be sure to join my email list at www.BoondocksBotanicals.com and be the first to hear about my latest book launches and regular free promotions.

Yours in Wellness,
Mary

Have you received your free eBook? If not, please take a quick moment to sign up for your gift:

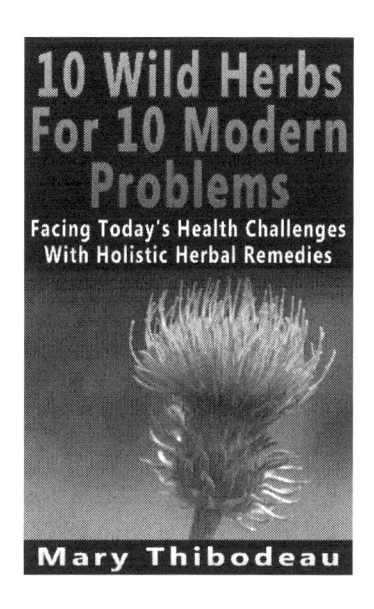

10 Wild Herbs For 10 Modern Problems
Facing Today's Health Challenges With Holistic Herbal Remedies
Mary Thibodeau

Have you always wanted to forage for medicine, but were afraid of picking the wrong plants or weren't sure how to use the herbs in the first place? Are you worried you won't have the time and know-how needed to get started?

I've written a detailed report for folks just like you – who have the intention and desire to forage for medicinal herbs, but who are in need of a quick and concise guide to start the journey.

So, for a limited time, this report will be free to my readers as a special thank you.

By downloading "Ten Wild Herbs for Ten Modern Problems" today, you'll enjoy an engaging beginner's guide to ten common medicinal herbs found in the wild, and how they can benefit your health.

You can get your free copy at:
www.BoondocksBotanicals.com.

Thank you and enjoy!

More Books by Mary Thibodeau
(Can be found at Amazon.com)

Herbal 1st Aid Hacks: 25 Herbal Remedies for First Aid and Healthy Living

Herbal Medicine First Aid Kit

Migraine: Natural Treatment and Prevention

Immune System Boosters: How to Naturally Boost Your Immune System and Stay Healthy All Year Long

Healing Lyme Disease Naturally

Cleanse: Holistic Strategies for Reducing Your Body's Chemical Load

Ten Wild Herbs for Ten Modern Problems

The Home Herbalism Companion

---

[i] http://www.greenmedinfo.com/blog/eating-flaxseed-may-reduce-breast-cancer-mortality-70

[ii] http://umm.edu/health/medical/altmed/herb/garlic

Made in the USA
Columbia, SC
30 November 2022